Her
HORMONE
Handbook
for Women

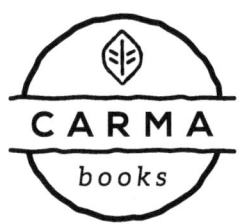

'A conscious approach to health & wellness'

carmabooks.com

You are invited to to join our **Free Book Club** mailing list. Sign up via our website to receive **special offers** and **free for a limited time** Health & Wellness eBooks!

Herbal HORMONE Handbook
for Women

Carmen Reeves

Copyright © 2015 Carma Books

All rights reserved. No part of this publication may be reproduced, distributed, or transmitted in any form or by any means, including photocopying, recording, or other electronic or mechanical methods, without the prior written permission of the publisher.

Disclaimer

This book provides general information and extensive research regarding health and related subjects. The information provided in this book, and in any linked materials is for informational purposes only, and is not intended to be construed as medical advice. Speak with your physician or other healthcare professional before taking any nutritional or herbal supplements. There are no 'typical' results from the information provided - as individuals differ, the results will differ. Before considering any guidance from this book, please ensure you do not have any underlying health conditions which may interfere with the suggested healing methods. If the reader or any other person has a medical concern or pre-existing condition, he or she should consult with an appropriately licensed physician or healthcare professional. Never disregard professional medical advice or delay in seeking it because of something you have read in this book or in any linked materials. The reader assumes the risk and full responsibility for all actions, and the author or publisher will not be held liable for any loss or damage that may result from the information presented in this publication.

Carma Books
carmabooks.com

hello@carmabooks.com

CONTENTS

INTRODUCTION

Bringing Natural Balance To Your Life 8

What Are Hormones and Why Are They Vital? 9
What Causes Hormonal Imbalance? 10
Common Signs and Symptoms 11
Diagnosing Hormonal Imbalance 12
Conventional and Alternative Treatments 13
General Lifestyle Tips to Enhance Hormonal Regulation 13

CHAPTER 1

Addressing Hormonal Imbalance, Gland by Gland 17

Hypothalamus 17
Pituitary Gland 18
Thyroid 19
Adrenal Glands 20
Pancreas 21
Ovaries 21
Pineal Gland 22

CHAPTER 2

Moods and Anxiety: Addressing Hormonal Fluctuations 24

Anxiety 25
Stress 26
Mood Swings & Irritability 27

Depression 28
Mental Foginess 29

CHAPTER 3
Normalizing Menstruation 31

Irregular Cycle 31
PMS 32
Cramps and Pain 33
Heavy Flow 34
Insomnia 35
Headaches 36

CHAPTER 4
Hormones and Diet Related Challenges 38

Weight Gain 39
Cravings 39
Water Retention 40
Bloating 41
Insulin Resistance 43
Digestive Problems 44

CHAPTER 5
Hormonal Health During Pregnancy and Childbirth 46

Nausea 46
Breast Pain & Tenderness 47
Labor Support 48
Postpartum Depression 49

CHAPTER 6
Perimenopause & Menopause 51

Irregular Periods 51
Hot Flashes & Night Sweats 52
Low Libido 53
Vaginal Dryness 54

CHAPTER 7
Other Common Hormonal Symptoms 56

Fatigue 56
Acne 57
Body Odor & Perspiration 58
Withdrawal From Birth Control Pills 59
Fibroids 61
Breast Cysts & Lumpiness 62
PCOS and Fertility 63
Endometriosis 64
Cervical Dysplasia 65

THANK YOU 67

A WORD FROM THE PUBLISHER 68

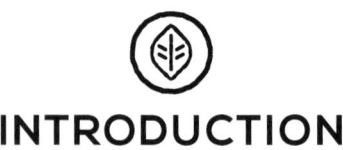

INTRODUCTION

Bringing Natural Balance to Your Life

Congratulations for purchasing the *Herbal Hormone Handbook for Women* and embarking on your journey to achieve natural hormonal balance. Hormonal health in women is often left unrecognized and ignored until adverse symptoms appear. By learning about our endocrine system and all that our hormones do, we can begin to nourish and tend our bodies holistically, thus getting to the root of the imbalance before it negatively affects our health. By reading this book you will learn exactly how to care for your body through the means of herbs, supplements and lifestyle choices, so that your hormones are balanced and your endocrine system can function optimally.

Having researched and experimented with herbalism for over ten years, I have seen the dramatic effects that simple, plant-based remedies and lifestyle changes can make to our overall health. Our current medical system is symptom driven; little action is taken in prevention until distinct symptoms arise, and the actions taken are often harsh, and at times, unnecessary. Synthetic hormones and other medications (with their various side effects) are usually the normal course of hormone imbalance treatment in conventional medicine. But, there is an alternate way to treat and help prevent hormonal issues before they worsen – a way that gently encourages improved physical function and allows you feel better without drugs or surgery. Isn't your body worth it?

You might be wondering why you are unable to lose weight, why you feel persistent low energy, or why you feel anxious or stressed. It may not always be obvious that our hormones are out of balance and could be the cause of our bothersome symptoms. You may be relieved to learn that there are ways to detect hormonal imbalances and address them with simple, effective strategies. To find out more about normalizing hormonal challenges and treating them with natural remedies, I invite you to continue reading this practical handbook, which outlines how to recognize an imbalance, and most importantly, how to make positive changes toward achieving hormonal harmony.

What are Hormones and Why are They Vital?

Hormones are a set of internally secreted compounds produced in the endocrine glands. They are transported to specific receptors cells in the organs and tissues throughout our bodies and will stimulate those cells into action when ordered by our brain. While many cells are exposed to the hormone being secreted, only certain "target cells" have the correct receptors to respond to the signal being sent. Hormones are responsible for coordinating complex body processes such as ***growth, fertility, reproduction*** and ***metabolism***. They also are an integral part of our immune system and they enable us to manage stress.

Because of their effect on so many essential bodily processes, hormones are vital to a functioning woman's body. Without hormones our bodies wouldn't grow when needed, or reach important life stages such as puberty and menopause. With no hormones our bodies would not be able to metabolize our food to create energy, signal our bodies to stop eating when satiated or react to stress and disease. Taking care to manage our hormone levels is a key to our overall health and staying healthy and balanced.

What Causes Hormonal Imbalance?

When we talk about hormonal imbalance it's important to distinguish between naturally occurring hormonal fluctuations and lifestyle associated symptoms. A woman goes through many times of change hormonally throughout her life, including the onset of menstruation, pregnancy, and menopause. These are natural changes in which our hormones play an important part. It has become a common belief that these bodily changes are the actual causes of hormonal imbalance, but in reality our hormones are acting specifically to honor and affect our body's necessary and normal changes. Adverse symptoms such as painful cramping and severe mood swings are not part of the normal hormonal process, but are signals that our health itself is compromised.

Our lifestyle plays a huge part in meeting the needs of our bodies as they go through essential hormonal changes. If we are overweight, over stressed, under exercised, exposed to harmful toxins and not getting regular sleep or proper nutrition, we are making it harder for our endocrine system to work and throwing our delicate hormonal balance off track. By understanding the needs of our bodies and encouraging the hormonal changes that are natural to women, we are better able to go through normal fluctuations without the negative symptoms often associated with them.

Common Signs and Symptoms of Hormonal Imbalance

Some symptoms of hormonal imbalance, such as hot flashes, heavy periods and PMS are easy to diagnose. Others are subtler and it may be harder to pinpoint their cause, like weight gain, cravings, anxiety, insomnia and digestive problems. For purposes of clarity the following breakdown into groups of symptoms has been created for easy reference. Each symptom will be discussed in detail in the following chapters. It's important to remember that many of these symptoms are not the natural course as is often assumed, but many of these problems can be avoided by caring for your body with diet, herbs and lifestyle enhancements.

- **Mood Fluctuations** – Anxiety, stress, mood swings and irritability, depression, mental fogginess

- **Menstruation** – Irregular cycle, PMS, cramps and pain, heavy flow, insomnia, headaches

- **Diet Related** – Weight gain, cravings, water retention, bloating, insulin resistance, digestive issues

- **Pregnancy and Childbirth** – Nausea, breast pain and tenderness, labor support, postpartum depression

- **Perimenopause and Menopause** – Irregular periods, hot flashes, night sweats, low libido, vaginal dryness

- **Other Common Symptoms** – Fatigue, acne, body odor and perspiration, withdrawal from birth control pills, fibroids, breast cysts, PCOS and fertility, endometriosis, cervical dysplasia

Many of the symptoms listed above are indicative of different types of imbalances, during various stages of the female body's life. This book will comprehensively cover a range of issues from adolescence to menopause and try to address each challenge.

Diagnosing Hormonal Imbalance

Being aware of the common symptoms of hormonal imbalance is the first step in enacting positive change. Visiting your doctor or alternative healthcare practitioner for a consultation will help you find out what exactly is going on. By administering a simple saliva test, your physician will be better able to determine the problem. Saliva tests have been used reliably for decades in determining the level of hormones including Cortisol, Estrogen, Progesterone and Testosterone in the tissues. This simple test will quickly establish the level of these hormones on a cellular level. It is also recommended to have a comprehensive blood test prior to a saliva test in order to rule out symptoms caused by other underlying factors or nutritional deficiencies.

Conventional and Alternative Treatments for Hormonal Imbalance

Conventional treatment of hormonal challenges centers around symptom-suppressing medications and surgeries, and does not consider the whole body in treating the root of the problem. For example, many young women with heavy bleeding during their periods are prescribed oral contraceptives as a solution. While taking the pill has been shown to reduce bleeding, cramps, PMS symptoms and acne breakouts, the list of possible side effects is lengthy. Some females will experience breast tenderness, vaginal discharge, nausea and headaches while those with previous cardiovascular disorders are at even more risk. Women over 35 and smokers are most at risk while taking oral contraceptives. The herbal and lifestyle tips included in this book do not simply mask the symptom while exposing us to dangerous side effects, but act gently to help your body put itself back into balance.

General Lifestyle Tips to Enhance Hormonal Imbalance

While herbal compounds and nutritional supplements can add accompanying support and nourishment to your endocrine system, there are many aspects of our lifestyle that can have a profound effect on our hormones. Below are some of the more common ways to complement your herbal and dietary program with hormonal balancing lifestyle improvements.

Eat a Diet Low in Refined Fat and High in Fruits and Vegetables

Eliminating or reducing polyunsaturated, refined and saturated fats (which have been linked to cell mutation and the slowing of metabolic processes), while at the same time emphasizing a diet heavy with whole plants, has been shown to have a positive effect on hormonal balance.

On a high fat diet, blood levels of hormones like estrogen are increased unnaturally. The production of estrogen, progesterone and prolactin can be normalized with a low fat, high plant fiber diet, and it is important to omit or limit fats from animal sources and refined fats such as vegetable oils, canola oil, soybean oil or other chemically altered fats. Dairy, whether conventional or organic, comes from pregnant and lactating cows with fluctuating hormones that have been shown to disrupt our own hormonal balance. Other dietary stressors, which may worsen symptoms, include alcohol, refined sugar and caffeine.

Avoid Known Endocrine Disruptors

This group of chemicals can mimic the body's hormones causing interference with our natural hormonal system and they can have the potential to produce adverse effects on our reproductive, developmental, neurological and immune systems. Some of the more common endocrine disruptors include **BPA**, a #7 plastic found in canned foods; **Dioxin**, which is commonly part of our food supply and which can be minimized by eating fewer animal products and more organic produce; **Atrazine**, an herbicide used widely for corn crops and often found in drinking water; and **Phthalates**, a #3 plastic found in body care products, often described only as "fragrance" in the ingredients. Unfortunately there are many others and an in-depth look into endocrine disruptors may be needed when all other lifestyle, nutritional and herbal aspects have already been addressed and hormonal imbalance continues.

Get Enough Sleep
The bad news is that getting too little sleep, 4-6 or less hours a night, has been shown repeatedly to adversely affect our endocrine system, stimulating abnormal elevations of Ghrelin (which stimulates hunger) and Cortisol (associated with stress, exercise and insulin production), while decreasing the amount of Leptin secretions (which signal satiety to our body). The good news is that these abnormalities can quickly be reversed by getting 8-10 hours of sleep per night, or by taking naps when needed.

Exercise Regularly
By exercising for 30 minutes a day for 3-5 days per week, we can cause positive effects to our endocrine system. Aerobic and strengthening workouts stimulate Human Growth Hormone (HGH), which while we are young helps with our development and once full grown continues to assist in building muscle mass, strengthening bones and metabolizing fat. PMS symptoms may be reduced as well with a similar exercise regimen, lessening cramps and mood swings. Many menopausal

symptoms are lessened with continued workouts and strengthening exercises.

Avoid Crash Diets
When dieting to lose weight quickly by focusing solely on calories, carbohydrates or weight loss, we are setting ourselves up for failure. Studies have shown that our hormones react to rapid weight loss by holding onto fat and slowing down our metabolism for a year or more after the weight is lost. By eating plentiful fruits, vegetables and whole grains, exercising moderately and losing weight gradually (with the focus on feeling healthier), our body's hormonal reaction will gently stabilize, resulting in a decrease of signals to crave unhealthy foods.

A steady and moderate intake of whole food carbohydrates is essential for our bodies to feel energized and regulate appetite control. A diet very low in carbohydrates may trigger thyroid issues, cause chronic inflammation, and can lead to an elevation of stress hormones.

For further support through this process, you may track your nutrients with an online food and exercise tracker such as *cronometer.com*. This type of application allows you to see exactly what nutrients you are consuming (or lacking), how many calories you are taking in (to ensure you're eating enough), and even lets you log your physical activity so you can regulate a slow, gradual weight loss. When consistently eating healthfully and keeping your hormones in check, your body *will* ultimately meet a healthy body weight.

CHAPTER 1

Addressing Hormonal Imbalance, Gland by Gland

This chapter is dedicated to giving you a key understanding of the value of each gland, a description of the hormones associated with it, the symptoms that may appear in the case of an imbalance, and suggestions for alternative, gentle treatments.

Hypothalamus

The Hypothalamus, located at the base of the brain, helps control the Pituitary Gland, which in turns regulates much of the endocrine system. The Hypothalamus regulates our secretions of Leptin and Ghrelin, which control our appetite. It is also responsible for producing thyrotropin-releasing hormone and release-inhibiting hormone and is primarily responsible for regulating hunger, thirst, blood temperature and nerve centers.

Symptoms of Imbalance:
Depression, headaches, fatigue, mental slowing, weight fluctuations, menstrual changes, dizziness, chills.

Natural Treatments:
Herbs: Maca Root

Supplements: B Vitamins

Lifestyle Adjustments:
Stress relieving activities like meditation, deep breathing and exercise, rest, limiting processed sugars.

Pituitary Gland

Otherwise knows and "The Master Gland" the Pituitary Gland is extremely important because of its relation to other glands in the body. Located near the optic nerves, it helps regulate the production of growth hormones, thyroid-stimulation hormone, adrenocorticotrophic hormone, and anti-diuretic hormone. When the pituitary gland is out of balance, tumors may develop which can result in excess hormones being made or a decrease in production. Usually these tumors are non-cancerous.

Symptoms of Imbalance:
Headaches, vision problems, nausea, weakness, unexplained weight loss or gain, feeling cold, irregular periods.

Natural Treatments:
Herbs: Chaste Tree Berry, Astragalus, Licorice

Supplements: B-12 injections

Lifestyle Adjustments:
Cutting out alcohol and tobacco products, increasing exercise and adopting healthier eating habits incorpo-

rating more fresh fruits and vegetables.

Thyroid

Located on the lower part of our neck, in front of our windpipe, the thyroid regulates our metabolism and body temperature. It also controls growth and development throughout our life and when we are young affects brain development. The thyroid secretes many hormones, most of which are grouped under the name, Thyroid Hormones.

Symptoms of Imbalance:
Dry skin, brittle nails, numbness or tingling in extremities, constipation, abnormal menstruation, joint pain, thinning hair, fatigue, weight fluctuation and anxiety.

Natural Treatments:
Herbs: Ashwagandha, Bladderwack, Echinacea

Supplements: Kelp, Iodine
(If you require a comprehensive iodine protocol, be sure to work closely with an iodine-literate practitioner)

Lifestyle Adjustments:
Regular, low fat meals rich in fruits and vegetables, regular sleeping patterns, strength training and yoga.

Adrenal Glands

Another essential body system, the Adrenals are responsible for regulating our blood sugar, mineral content, digestive functioning, energy levels and stress monitoring hormones. Located atop our kidneys, the adrenals secrete two major hormones, adrenaline and cortisol, which control our reactions to short-term stress and acute stress, respectively. From the list of symptoms below it is clear that the Adrenals have profound effects on our health.

Symptoms of Imbalance:
Extreme fatigue, irritability, mental fogginess, sleep disorders, food addictions, PMS, diabetes, headaches, chronic low blood pressure, weight fluctuations (particularly around midsection), hot flashes and memory loss.

Natural Treatments:
Herbs: Ashwagandha, Licorice, Gingko, Rhodiola

Supplements: B5, B6, B12, Vitamin C, Magnesium, Probiotics (dairy free), Sea Salt

Lifestyle Adjustments:
Regular meals, especially an early breakfast, plenty of sleep and rest, stress reducing habits like meditating, exercising and deep breathing, reduction or elimination of caffeine and refined sugars.

If you suspect you have Adrenal Fatigue, you may benefit from my comprehensive and holistic self-help guide: *Adrenal Fatigue: Cure it Naturally (A Fresh Approach)*.

Pancreas

Sitting across the back of our abdomen, behind the stomach, is the Pancreas, which works in two important ways. Its first major role involves releasing digestive enzymes needed to help convert starches into simple sugars. The second role is to control blood sugar by secreting the hormones insulin and glucagon.

Symptoms of Imbalance:
Abdominal pain, nausea, vomiting, diarrhea, bloating and fever.

Natural Treatments:
Herbs: Turmeric, Ginger

Supplements: Grape Seed Extract, Curcumin

Lifestyle Adjustments:
Keeping well hydrated, a low fat diet, avoiding alcohol, eating regular, smaller meals throughout the day instead of 3 large meals.

Ovaries

The Ovaries are situated at the opposite ends of our pelvic wall, on either side of the uterus. There they help maintain a woman's reproductive health. They produce two major groups of hormones, estrogens and progesterone.

Symptoms of Imbalance:
Pain and tenderness or sore/burning sensation in lower abdomen, increased facial hair growth and irregular periods (many times ovarian cysts go unnoticed, without symptoms, so it may be of benefit to have regular exams).

Natural Treatments:
Herbs: Borage Oil, Evening Primrose Oil

Supplements: Flax Seed Oil (or regularly consuming ground flaxseeds in smoothies or salads)

Lifestyle Adjustments:
Healthy whole food fats in the diet such as nuts and seeds, minimizing or eliminating meat and dairy, stress reduction techniques like meditation, deep breathing, yoga and exercise.

Pineal Gland

The Pineal Gland was the last gland to be discovered and is still somewhat of a mystery. Often referred to as the "Third Eye" this gland is right in the center of the brain and produces the hormone melatonin, which is responsible for maintaining our circadian rhythm, otherwise know as our biological clock. The Pineal Gland also maintains appropriate levels of gonadotrophins, which are essential to the function of the ovaries.

Symptoms of Imbalance:
Sleep disorders, breast soreness, alcohol cravings and menstrual irregularities.

Natural Treatments:
Herbs: Oregano Oil, Neem Extract

Supplements: Kelp, Iodine
(If you require a comprehensive iodine protocol, be sure to work closely with an iodine-literate practitioner)

Lifestyle Adjustments:
Reduce exposure to artificial light, don't stay up or work late at night if possible, reduce stress and cut out excess refined sugars, reduce fluoride consumption (in water) and increase intake of organic produce.

CHAPTER 2

Mood and Anxiety:
Addressing Hormonal Fluctuations

If only women could lead a stress-free life. Not only are we faced with societal pressures and stresses – most of us were raised to suppress our negative emotions, or were taught to 'learn to live with it'. Not addressing and dealing with our feelings only increases our anxiety.

Our adrenals were designed to deal with 'fight or flight' stress, or quick elevations of needed hormones to get us through a drastic situation. But the stress of modern society pushes the limits of our adrenals by providing us with a multiple of daily stressful situations - much more than the adrenals are designed to handle. Prolonged stress will wear down our adrenals and cause many symptoms like weight gain, blood sugar imbalances, depression and memory loss.

To address this serious lack of emotional stability and hormonal balance and give extra support to our adrenals, it's smart to look at all aspects of our lives. We know that eating a low-fat diet rich with fruits and vegetables plays a part, and we know that yoga, aerobic exercise and strength training all make us feel better in many ways. We cannot forget our emotional selves and it's important to learn ways to process negative emotions and celebrate our selves.

Anxiety:
Remedies to Reduce Nervousness

Though anxiety often is associated with emotions, it also manifests itself in physical symptoms; feelings of panic can cause shortness of breath, a pounding heartbeat, and lack of focus. Anxiety often is the result of repressed emotions and prolonged stress and can be worse during a woman's hormonal fluctuations.

Herbs:
Passion Flower Tea - Used traditionally for anxiety, Passion Flower has gentle yet effective sedatives properties. Infuse 1 teaspoon of the dried herb per cup with boiling water, let sit off the heat for 10 minutes and drink, up to 4 cups per day. You may also take a Passion Flower tincture, putting 15 drops into your mouth 3 times per day. *(Do not use if you are pregnant or lactating, and consult your physician if you are on any anxiety medications)*

Supplements:
Magnesium - Moderns diets, with refined and processed foods, are virtually devoid of this powerful, calming mineral. Take 400mg per day for anxiety support.

Lifestyle Tips:
Because repression of negative emotions is common in our society and can cause anxiety, finding a way to take care of our emotional side is imperative. ***Emotion Freedom Technique*** is a process using tapping/

acupressure with positive affirmations to help calm and relax our bodies and minds. A variety of simple how-to videos can be found online.

Stress:
Natural Relief Techniques

The amount of stress we are faced with in daily life is far more than our bodies were intended to deal with. In a stressful situation, our hormones react by secreting more cortisol for a quick release of energy. Nature designed this system for 'fight or flight' situations and not day-to-day activities. This overload of cortisol and our bodies' reactions can even make our stress worse.

Herbs:
Ashwaganda - Otherwise known as 'Indian Ginseng', Ashwagandha naturally lowers cortisol levels and supports our immune system. Take 500mg per day.

Supplements:
B Complex Vitamins - B vitamins help keep our stress levels neutral and act as a general tonic to the nervous system. Since they usually include Vitamin C, a B Complex supplement also supports the immune system.

Lifestyle Tips:
One of the best ways to relieve stress is through **body contact**. Snuggling, hugging, holding hands and massage are all ways to send calming and comforting messages to the brain.

Mood Swings and Irritability:
Finding Balance

Most women have experienced mood swings and irritability at some point during their lifetime – often during hormonal fluctuations. Overreacting in situations or exhibiting inappropriate (and unusual to you) responses to life's occurrences may signal you are suffering from mood swings and irritability.

Herbs:
Evening Primrose Oil - With it's high content of the essential fatty acids, Gamma Linolenic Acid (GLA), Evening Primrose Oil offers an alternative way to get the GLA's necessary for hormonal balance without including high-allergen foods such as soy and dairy. Take 500mg twice per day.

Supplements:
Vitamin D - Also called the sunshine vitamin, Vitamin D has been shown to prevent mood instability. Though we get this nutrient via the sun, folks living in wintery places are almost always deficient without supplementation. 2000IU per day is recommended.

Lifestyle Tips:
Diet is probably the easiest way to positively effect mood swings and irritability. Cutting out refined sugars, processed foods and common allergens like dairy, soy and gluten, and replacing them with an abundance of fruit, vegetables, beans, nuts, seeds and whole grains helps your endocrine system work properly and works to normalize mood swings and irritability.

Depression: Tips to Help Lift your Mood

One in eight women suffer from some level of depression. The causes vary from social pressures, to nutritional deficiencies to hormonal imbalances. Since depression itself has an impact on every area of a woman's life, it's important to address depression with a holistic approach.

Herbs:
Saint John's Wort Capsules - Saint John's Wort is a powerful yet gentle nervine, anti-depressant and anti-inflammatory herb supporting the nervous system and often used to help treat depression. 300mg, 2-3 times per day is recommended. *(Saint John's Wort interferes with some pharmaceuticals thus it is imperative to check with your physician before taking this herb. Do not use this herb if you are taking any pharmaceutical anti-depressants.)*

Supplements:
Folic Acid - It has been shown that those low in folic acid do not respond as well to treatments for depression. Supplementing with folic acid aids in the effectiveness of antidepressants. 400-600 micrograms is the standard daily dosage.

Lifestyle Tips:
Strength Training, also called weight training or resistance training, has been shown repeatedly to improve sleep, give more energy, enhance metabolism and give the person exercising a higher self image. With the increased heart pumping and endorphin boosting

that strength training can provide, it is worth it to start a program to help lessen depression symptoms. Always check with your health care practitioner before starting a program.

Mental Fogginess:
Ways to Improve Mental Clarity

Mental Fogginess can be apparent in women who feel confusion, lack of focus or forgetfulness and can certainly interfere with daily life. Natural remedies that focus on our nervous system can help bring clarity.

Herbs:
Gingko Biloba - Known as the oldest living tree species, Gingko Biloba had been used extensively for memory improvement. This herb improves blood circulation, enhances oxygen utilization and helps your brain function better. 240mg per day for up to 10 weeks is the standard dose.

Supplements:
B12 - It's very common to be deficient in B12, which is essential to healthy nerve cells and energy production. 2.4 mc daily is recommended for adults, 2.6 for pregnant women, 2.8 for lactating women and 25-100 for women over 50 years of age.

Lifestyle Tips:
Avoid Neurotoxins and Eat Berries - Eliminating all toxic additives such as MSG and artificial sweeteners will go a long way in ridding your diet of harmful and

interfering neurotoxins. Also adding in copious amounts of antioxidant-rich berries (strawberries, blueberries, raspberries, blackberries, etc) will support neuron function and protect brain cells.

CHAPTER 3

Normalizing Menstruation

Probably every woman has experienced either heavy menstruation, missed periods or painful or irritating symptoms during their regular cycle at some point in their life. The monthly changes our bodies go through depend on a very delicate and easily disrupted hormonal system. Most of these symptoms can be reduced and improved with adjustments to diet, exercise habits and stress reduction techniques.

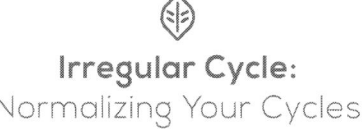

Irregular Cycle:
Normalizing Your Cycles

It is a sign of imbalance if we miss periods (unless pregnant or going through menopause), or have them too often. Bringing our bodies back into balance by adjusting our diet and lifestyle habits will help our cycles become more regular.

Herbs:

Vitex Tincture (Chaste Tree Berry) - Nicknamed "The Women's Herb", Vitex gently regulates our Pituitary Gland (the master gland) and helps bring hormonal levels to where they should be. Take 40 drops of the tincture per day. This herb works as a tonic and may take 3-6 months before its balancing effects are felt.

Supplements:
Walnuts for EFA's - Just 3 tablespoons of walnuts per day contributes 181% of your Omega-3 Fatty Acids and 70% Omega-6 Fatty Acids. Sufficient EFA's in the diet are essential in regulating hormonal levels.

Lifestyle Tips:
Ditch the Coffee and Switch to Green Tea - Because coffee is known to affect hormonal secretions, switching to green tea, which is high in antioxidants and Vitamin C, will give you a nutritive way to start your day (whilst supporting your hormones).

PMS:
Reducing Symptoms

Before each period, our bodies are busy increasing levels of estrogen and decreasing levels of progesterone. When lifestyle habits negatively affect our health, PMS symptoms like irritability, breast tenderness and headaches may worsen. Bringing our bodies back into balance by adjusting our diet and lifestyle habits will help regulate our hormonal secretions so that our cycles become more regular and PMS symptoms are reduced.

Herbs:
Burdock Root Tea - Because of Burdock Root's anti-inflammatory actions and its small amount of natural plant steroids, it helps improve the metabolism of estrogen thus lessening hormonal symptoms during PMS. One cup of the tea daily is the standard dosage.

Supplements:

Magnesium Citrate Powder - Supplementing with Magnesium has been shown to decrease symptoms of PMS. 2 teaspoons in water per day is the standard dose.

Lifestyle Tips:

Eliminate Refined Flours - During the 'refining' process so many nutrients are lost: calcium, magnesium, iron, magnesium and EFA's – all of which are essential to hormonal health and balance. Switching to nutrient rich whole grains, fruits and vegetables will increase your body's overall nutrient base making it easier for your hormones to stay in balance.

Cramps:
Decreasing Menstrual Pain

Menstrual cramping can vary in degrees; from slight discomfort to severe pain that interrupts your daily activities. It is caused by uterine contractions that when too strong, constrict blood vessels and cut off oxygen supply, and usually signals over production of prostaglandin. Cramps should not be considered normal and there are many ways to reduce and eliminate this monthly bane.

Herbs:

Red Raspberry Leaf - Because of it's high nutrient content (including 54% of your daily calcium) and it's reputation as the best uterine tonic, a cup of Red Raspberry Leaf Tea taken each day (or a daily capsule) helps reduce pelvic muscle spasms, nausea, and replenishes your body much needed nutrients in a gentle, plant-based form.

Supplements:
Calcium Citrate - Since Calcium is responsible for maintaining muscle tone, including that of your uterus, it makes a great addition to your daily nutrient regimen. 500mg per day or one large salad with dark leafy greens each day is recommended.

Lifestyle Tips:
Yoga – Various yoga poses specifically designed for menstrual cramping can help effectively relieve and reduce pain. Such poses include: Janu Sirsasana A *(head-to-knee forward bend)*, Pasasana *(noose pose)*, Ustrasana *(camel pose)*, and Supta Padangusthasana *(reclining big toe pose)*.

Heavy Flow:
Regulating Your Period

Abnormally heavy menstruation, also called Menorrhagia, signals an imbalance of our estrogen and progesterone hormonal secretions. An appointment with your gynecologist will ensure that heavy bleeding isn't a symptom of another disorder. The following tips are for those with heavy periods caused by hormonal imbalance.

Herbs:
Ginger Root - Shown in several studies to have dramatic effects on menstrual flow, ginger also helps

with pain and inflammation making it the perfect herb for heavy periods. 1-3mg per day is the regularly dosage.

Supplements:

Floradix Iron Supplement - This natural, plant-based iron supplement helps restore the iron levels in women with heavy blood loss, who may be suffering from anemia. 10mg of the liquid per day provides about 60% of your recommended daily iron, plus all of your B vitamins.

Lifestyle Tips:

Keep Hydrated - Drinking enough water is always important, but during our periods, because of the loss of fluids, becomes even more essential. 6-8 cups of filtered water per day goes a long way in helping your body do its job. Eating a plant-rich diet full of fruits and vegetables also provides your body with extra water and hydration, along with fiber, vitamins and minerals.

Insomnia:
Readying Your Body for Sleep

About 67% of women have reported sleep issues during their menstrual cycle. This often happens right before your period starts, as levels of progesterone drop and the sedative properties of that hormone decrease. If the drop is too severe, a sleep disruption may be the result. The following tips can help your body get ready for sleep while minimizing the hormonal change.

Herbs:

Chamomile - With its sedative, anti-inflammatory and muscle relaxing properties, Chamomile Tea is the perfect herb for helping ready your body for a restful night of sleep. To make a strong dose (and not drink too much before bed) use 2-3 teabags of Chamomile Tea in a mug and fill about to two thirds with boiling water. Cover and steep for 15 minutes and drink an hour or two before bed each night.

Supplements:

Wild Yam Cream - Wild Yam is a natural progesterone regulator. A small amount can be massaged until thoroughly absorbed into your chest, abdomen, inner arms or thighs nightly.

Lifestyle Tips:

Create a Sleep Ready Environment - Make it dark and quiet. Use a sleep mask or dark curtains if necessary and turn your clock away from you. Keep your electronic devices out of your bedroom. If you live in a noisy neighborhood, consider a small fan for white noise. Try to keep a regular sleep schedule and a predictable bedtime.

Hormonal Headaches:
Best Tips to Treat Headaches Naturally

When our estrogen levels drop before menstruation, many women experience a headache, sometimes even a migraine. By paying attention to our bodies and seeking holistic solutions, these hormonal drops become less severe.

Herbs:
Vitex Tincture - Because of its ability to help regulate levels of estrogen and progesterone, Vitex has been shown repeatedly to help with hormonal headaches. Standard does is 40 drops per day and it may take a few months for results to start kicking in.

Supplements:
CoEnzyme Q10 (CoQ10) - This enzyme supports both cell function and biological processes like muscle contractions and has been shown in studies to significantly reduce hormonal headaches. Take 150-300mg per day.

Lifestyle Tips:
Routine - Your body will love you right back if you make the effort to consume regular meals throughout the day, plus a regular exercise and sleep routine that you will stick with. A routine of daily meditation will also help. Regular habits will allow you to function with familiarity and calm, helping stabilize hormonal fluctuations.

CHAPTER 4

Hormones and Diet Related Challenges

The relationship between hormones and poor diet is like a double-edged sword – you simply can't achieve hormonal balance if you eat a terrible diet; and you can't regulate bodyweight without balanced hormones. Hormonal health relies on proper nutrition. Lack of essential nutrients will have a negative effect on the physiological processes that hormones regulate. By addressing the ways we obtain these nutrients, and minimizing stress, our bodies will be better able to achieve hormonal harmony.

Weight Gain:
Allowing Your Body to Heal

Eliminating meals and slashing calories will signal to our bodies that food is scarce, thus starting the biological process of storing fat and slowing our metabolism. Eating the foods that we need, setting up regular eating habits and initiating a strength training program will allow our bodies to self regulate and achieve a healthy bodyweight.

Herbs:
Dandelion - All parts of this powerful plant have a multitude of medicinal properties. The short list

includes: slows of digestion (making satiety last longer), is full of vitamins and minerals including 111% Vitamin A and 32% Vitamin C, is a natural liver cleanser and contains a good source of fiber and natural sodium. Teas or tinctures made with the flowers, leaves and/or roots are great, or you can easily pick and steam the young greens or eat them raw when available.

Supplements:
Cinnamon - By boosting glucose metabolism and enhancing blood sugar regulation, Cinnamon makes a perfect addition to your weight control plan. 1g per day of powdered Cinnamon is the standard dosage.

Lifestyle Tips:
Eliminate Refined Carbs and Try Strength Training - Consuming 'foods' with heavily refined flours and processed sugars can completely throw off our hormones. Without the fiber and nutrients attached (like in whole foods), these processed products leave our bodies lacking and confused. Get rid of sodas, artificial ingredients and highly processed packaged foods, and replace them with an abundance of fruits, vegetables, nuts, seeds and whole grains. In addition, a strength training program will assist you in your weight goals by building more muscle (which helps burns more fat!).

Cravings:
Curbing them Naturally

When we eat too much of the wrong foods our bodies become desensitized to our body's signals to stop eating.

When we restrict calories and skip meals we will only crave food more. Taking a moment to feel the craving, asking ourselves what we really need, and acting on it can play a part in reducing the effects cravings have on our eating habits.

Herbs:
Pine Nuts - High in Omega-6 Fatty Acids, pine nuts also increase the effectiveness of satiety hormones (signaling when we are full) and are an excellent source of protein and iron. A small handful as a supplement with a meal or in a homemade pesto may be eaten daily.

Supplements:
Chromium Picolinate - A naturally occurring mineral, Chromium has been shown to normalize glucose levels and curb appetite. 130mcg per day is the recommended dose.

Lifestyle Tips:
Take a Moment - When feeling a craving, pause for a moment. Sometimes our body is in need of water or stress relief rather than that greasy donut! Have a glass of water, go for a short walk, or take a moment for a cup of calming herbal tea. If you still feel hunger, have a nutritious, whole food snack or meal, and avoid processed foods.

Water Retention:
Balancing our Fluid Levels

When the ratio of sodium to water throughout our

body is too high, our kidneys react by retaining water and diluting the salt so it does not irritate our tissues. Ditching table salt and processed foods, which are extremely high in sodium, are the first steps in reducing water retention.

Herbs:
Parsley - Parsley is a natural and effective diuretic, promoting our water balance and enhancing urine elimination with its minerals and phytochemicals. A small amount each day in your salad, soup or smoothie is sufficient.

Supplements:
Quercetin – Because of its ability to stabilize small blood vessels, Quercetin helps to reduce fluid retention. 100mg per day is the standard dose. Brightly colored fruits and vegetables, and grains, also contain a natural source of Quercetin.

Lifestyle Tips:
Break a Sweat - When we exercise and sweat we are boosting our circulation and helping to get our fluids moving. This will aid in excess water elimination.

Bloating:
Simple Recipes for Reduction

It's common for women to experience abdominal bloating during the two weeks before menstruation. Rising hormone levels can often have an effect on the gastrointestinal tract, slowing down digestion and prolonging the time gas is moving through the system. Strategies to improve digestion, when combined with hormonal balancing remedies can improve this bothersome symptom.

Herbs:
Peppermint Tea - Drinking a cup of Peppermint tea has been shown to have a positive effect on bloating and pain due to gas. It's antispasmodic and relaxant properties target the GI tract while its volatile oils stimulate bile, which will enhance digestion. 1-3 cups per day can be used when abdominal pain is a problem.

Supplements:
Dandelion Greens - A mild diuretic is often prescribed by doctors to help with bloating. Unfortunately, pharmaceutical diuretics also leach potassium and have other side effects. Dandelion, once again, proves itself a perfect supplement: a gentle diuretic that's full of vitamins and minerals, including potassium. The dried, encapsulated herb can be taken 3 times per day.

Lifestyle Tips:
Bloating Exercise - Lie on your back and bring one leg up, lace your hands on that knee and bring the knee forward towards your face as far as you can, and hold for 20 seconds. Your other leg should be laying flat. Repeat on the other side and alternate 4 or 5 times until relief is felt.

Insulin Resistance:
Restoring our Bodies

This pre-diabetic symptom results from hormonal imbalance and sets up the body for greater risk of diabetes, obesity, heart disease, PCOS and breast cancer. The best strategies will include a combination of exercise and diet adjustments.

Herbs:
Fenugreek - Because of its ability to help slow down digestion and enhance the absorption of carbohydrates, a cup of Fenugreek tea each day is recommended.

Supplements:
Hemp Seed Oil - The cold pressed, unrefined seed oil of Hemp contains a ratio of Essential Fatty Acids (EFA's) that fits the needs of a human body (3:1 Omega-6 to Omega-3). EFA's stimulate fat burning and enhance insulin function. A few teaspoons a day in a smoothie, soup or salad will not only cover your daily EFA needs but also will provide you will an excellent source of protein and Vitamin E.

Lifestyle Tips:
Aerobic Exercise and Reduce Saturated Fat - Getting your heart pumping through regular aerobic exercise helps decrease the cells' resistance to insulin. 30 minutes a day of swimming, walking, running or biking is an important recommendation for insulin resistance. Also, reducing your saturated fat intake will ensure your insulin response is not hindered. By reducing the

amount of fat that enters our bloodstream, we allow our bodies to process natural sugars and carbohydrates more efficiently.

Digestive Problems:
Ways to Ease Digestion

Many women experience constipation or loose bowel movements around the time of their periods. If hormones are out of whack, digestion can be compromised. Keeping active and eating foods that promote digestion can assist.

Herbs:
Powdered Psyllium Seed - A tablespoon of Psyllium Seed in water, a smoothie or in your meal each day will enhance intestinal contractions thus speeding up digestion. With its excellent fiber content and soothing mucilage, this supplement works well for digestive issues.

Supplements:
Probiotics - Restoring our intestinal flora, especially to those who have undergone a round of antibiotics, will not only tone the digestive system, but also helps with immunity and has been shown to relieve other digestive diseases like irritable bowel syndrome. Opt for a dairy-free probiotic supplement or consume natural sources such as sauerkraut, kimchi or kombucha tea.

Lifestyle Tips:
Take a Walk and Add Fluids and Fiber - Walking

after a meal encourages digestion and relaxes the body. Even 10 to 15 minutes will be helpful. If you are already fit, more vigorous exercise may be in order, but wait until an hour after your meal. Extra fluids and fiber are vital for improved digestion. Raw fruits and vegetables are full of both, plus essential vitamins and minerals.

CHAPTER 5

Hormonal Health During Pregnancy and Childbirth

During pregnancy, labor and postpartem, our hormones are busy making all the essential physiological processes involved occur, producing a huge fluctuation in estrogen and progesterone. Other hormones like oxytocin, endorphins and adrenaline will also come into play throughout this time. Hormonal imbalance can lead to worsened symptoms, which often results in medical interventions. It is of upmost importance to keep hormones balanced during this time.

Nausea:
Finding Relief Naturally

About 75% of women experience some level of nausea (also referred to as 'morning sickness') during the first trimester of pregnancy. There are many ways to ease this symptom and help promote hormonal harmony at the same time.

Herbs:
Anise Tea - A natural stomachic, Anise Tea daily makes a refreshing, calming and soothing tonic to aid with digestion and nausea.

Supplements:

B6 - Taking a B6 supplement has been shown to improve nausea among pregnant women. A regular dose would be 25mg per day. It can also be found in many foods including bananas, nuts, green beans, carrots and potatoes.

Lifestyle Tips:

Take lots of Ginger and Eat Frequently - Because ginger has the power to neutralize acids and relaxes stomach issues, it makes a great pregnancy companion. Make a tea or include in your favorite recipes. Having an empty stomach can intensify the nausea. To help with this, keep a few nuts or whole grain crackers nearby for those nighttime bathroom trips and for when you first awake.

Breast Tenderness:
Alleviating Pain

Often an early symptom of pregnancy (can also occur during PMS) and linked with a rise in progesterone, breast pain and tenderness can vary in severity. A few comfort measures and plant-based therapies have been said to help reduce this symptom.

Herbs:

Stinging Nettle Tea - Traditionally used as a pregnancy tonic, Stinging Nettle supports the female reproductive system. Packed with minerals like iron and calcium, and vitamins E and K, Stinging Nettle Tea also acts a blood strengthener. Enjoy 1-3 cups per day.

Supplements:
Sea Kelp - With a naturally high content of iodine, Sea Kelp capsules provide an excellent antioxidant source for breast tissue support. 225mcg per day is the recommended dose.

Lifestyle Tips:
Reduce Processed Fat in Your Diet and Opt for Healthy Fats - Research has shown that a high fat diet raises estrogen levels – this unnatural altering of our hormonal secretions may be lessened by cutting out unhealthy fats (like fried foods, red meat and dairy) and adding in healthful fats like avocado, nuts and seeds.

Labor Support:
Aiding our Bodies

Highly medicalized births, which are so common in the western world, often lead to interventions that throw off the complex hormonal processes that occur during labor. Because stress and fear alone can cause alterations to the hormonal function, having the support of a mid-wife and a doula to advocate for your needs during labor will go a long way toward making you feel safe, relaxed and supported.

Herbs:
Raspberry Leaf Tea - This effective uterine tonic can be drunk to soothe and strengthen the uterus, and may lessen pain during contractions. During labor, an iced version with a little lemon will help restore necessary fluids and nutrients.

Supplements:
Love and Support - A loved one to provide gentle pressure to counter pain during labor, a sister to hold your hand, a birthing tub, the most loving, supportive people you know in the room with you – any of these things can relax your mind and body so labor can progress naturally and without fear.

Lifestyle Tips:
Get comfortable - Lying on your back on a hospital bed is not the most practical way to labor, it only makes it convenient for medical personnel. Using gravity makes sense: walk or move around as much as you can, relax on a yoga ball, or have someone hold you. Find the position for birthing that feels right to you.

Postpartem Depression:
Finding Support

Possibly due to the severe drop in estrogen and progesterone directly after birth, many women have strong mood swings and may experience insomnia or find it difficult to bond with their newborn. Fatigue, bodily changes, the stress of a complete life change and dramatic hormonal changes are to be expected. To minimize the effects of these challenges is essential during a woman's transition through this time.

Herbs:
Blessed Thistle Leaf Capsules - This intensely bitter herb stimulates gastric juices, acts as a mild diuretic, enhances liver function and is an overall uterine tonic

thus helping your body with this wondrous adjustment. 3 to 4 capsules daily is the standard dose.

Supplements:
Prenatal Vitamins - The same vitamins you've been taking during your pregnancy will continue to give you much needed nutrients, including folic acid, iron and many other vitamins and minerals. The same dosage can be used.

Lifestyle Tips:
Get Help, Say No, and Sing - When people ask you if they can help, take them up on it. But get help with housework and errands while you bond with your baby or rest. If you're not up for going out, don't. Stay home and rest as much as possible.

It has been shown in studies that singing to your baby not only relaxes you and your newborn, but it also provides a way to process emotions and it increases feelings of overall wellbeing.

CHAPTER 6

Perimenopause and Menopause

Because perimenopause refers to the time leading up to menopause, the symptoms of perimenopause and menopause are one and the same. Women can be in perimenopause anywhere from two to ten years. It is generally after 12 months with no menses that a woman is said to have reached menopause. Most of the symptoms can be reduced with herbals therapies, exercise and diet changes.

Irregular Periods:
Managing Changes

Often one of the first symptoms to show during perimenopause, many women will experience the absence of a period (or periods), a lengthening of the period's duration, or an increase in bleeding. It is a good time to start ways to accept menopause into your life, not as an annoyance but as an important stage.

Herbs:
Black Current Oil - This plant-based source of GLA's (omega-6 fatty acids) helps balance hormones during perimenopause and menopause, encouraging prostaglandin synthesis while stimulating our immune system and providing antioxidants. 1g per day is the

recommended dosage.

Supplements:
Black Cohosh - With its potent phytochemicals, Black Cohosh has been long used in Native American medicine to help tone the reproductive system, promote menstrual cycles, heal menstrual irregularities and encourage hormonal balance (from PMS through to menopausal symptoms). Take in supplement form or enjoy as a tea.

Lifestyle Tips:
Ditch Refined Sugar, Caffeine and Alcohol and Eat Lentils - If these three substances (refined sugar, caffeine and alcohol) are still in your diet by the time you reach perimenopause, your symptoms may be more severe than those who have forgone them. Consuming lentils offers your body a great source of iron, protein, B vitamins and fiber. This remarkable mix of nutrients has a stabilizing effect on blood sugar.

Hot Flashes and Night Sweats:
Minimizing Discomfort

A sudden rise in body temperature is a normal hormonal fluctuation that happens to many women during perimenopause and menopause. These hot flashes (or during sleep, night sweats) can occur with regularity, or with no warning at all and cause much discomfort. By the time we start experiencing menopausal symptoms, our adrenals, which take on a more active role during this time, may be already exhausted due to lifestyle habits and lack of proper nutrients. It's imperative during this time to eat a healthy diet and exercise to help minimize this symptom.

Herbs:
Dong Quai Capsules - This herb supports natural hormone balance and increases oxygen utilization. Take 3 capsules, 3 times per day. (Do not take if you have heavy bleeding)

Supplements:
Red Clover Capsules - Rich in phytoestrogens and isoflavones, red clover has been shown to gently support the regulation of hormones. 80mg per day is the standard dose.

Lifestyle Tips:
Exercise - At this point I must be sounding like a broken record, but several studies have shown that women who exercise regularly (30 minutes of aerobic exercise 3-5 times per week) experienced a significant decrease in hot flashes.

Low Libido:
Understanding the Reasons

Having a low sex drive during any stage of your adult life, including perimenopause and menopause, commonly signals other health issues. A history of medical diseases, prescriptions, alcohol, street drugs or smoking can adversely affect the hormones involved. Fatigue, another prevalent factor, is often present if the adrenals or thyroid are overtaxed. This new set of hormonal changes cannot function optimally if the body is unhealthy, so focusing on nutrition is essential to restoring sex drive. If a woman is experiencing pain due to vaginal dryness (addressed in the next section) this will also need to be treated.

Herbs:
Motherwort - Nourishing the heart and stimulating enhanced blood oxygenation, Motherwort herb is also uterine specific, acting as a thorough tonifier. 1-3 cups per day of the herbal tea, or 30 drops of a tincture would be the regular dose.

Supplements:
Maca Root - Sexual hormones need iodine and zinc to function properly and Maca Root, which is high in both, can assist. Take 4-6 capsules per day.

Lifestyle Tips:
Yoga - Most types of exercise have positive effect on self-esteem and energy levels. Regular yoga practice, in particular, can help improve sexual function and desire, as well as increasing flexibility to help improve your self-image and sex life.

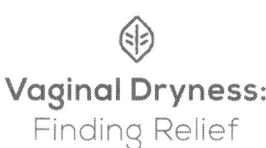

Vaginal Dryness:
Finding Relief

During the year surrounding menopause, one of many changes taking place to our reproductive system is the thinning of the vaginal walls and a reduction in their elasticity. For some this may not cause problems, but for others inflammation and dryness worsen the symptom making it uncomfortable or even painful, especially during sex. With a few simple supplements, a reduction in refined foods and exercise this symptom can be greatly reduced.

Herbs:
Comfrey Ointment - Offered in most natural food markets or online, a Comfrey Ointment applied directly will soothe the vaginal tissues and make them more flexible, strong and soft.

Supplements:
Vitamin E - An excellent supplement for dryness, Vitamin E can be taken daily in gel-caps or applied directly. 400-600mg per day is standard.

Lifestyle Tips:
Hydration and Coconut Oil - 2 quarts (2L) of filtered water daily will ensure your body has enough moisture. During intercourse, if lubrication is needed, coconut oil not only is plant-based and non-toxic, but has many soothing properties.

CHAPTER 7

The Road to Recovery

Some symptoms of hormonal balance come at different times in a woman's life and reproductive cycle. The following is a comprehensive look at some of the more common symptoms of hormonal imbalance.

Fatigue:
Supporting the Adrenals

The fact that adrenal fatigue has become so prevalent in modern society is a symptom itself of widespread nutritional deficiencies coupled with too much stress. Doing what we can to support and nourish our adrenals will help not only with fatigue; it can aid our metabolism, immunity and the many other body systems with which the adrenals are associated.

Herbs:
Rhidiola - Traditionally, Rhidiola has been used to enhance strength and endurance and reduce physical and mental fatigue by working to normalize bodily systems. The result is a body better able to adapt to stress. 100-400mg is the recommendation.

Supplements:
B-Complex - B vitamins are vital to the adrenal glands

many processes. 500mg per day is standard.

Lifestyle Tips:
Skip the High Glycemic Foods - Foods like white sugar and those made with refined flour quickly and unnaturally raise your blood sugar level because they are devoid of the fiber, vitamins and minerals in whole roods. Eliminating these foods will make a huge difference in the health of your adrenals.

Acne:
Ways to a Clearer Face

It is common for acne symptoms, which are inflammatory in nature, to worsen about a week before menstruation. Of the many hormonal symptoms, acne is one of the few that can actually affect a woman's self-esteem, so it is important to use hormonal balancing measures and healthy tips to reduce this symptom.

Herbs:
Clove Essential Oil in Apricot Kernel Carrier Oil - Clove oil contains anti-inflammatory, antioxidant, anti-bacterial and anti-fungal properties. By adding a few drops to a tablespoon of Apricot Kernel Oil and dabbing the mixture directly onto facial pimples 1-3 times per day, the clove oil can go to work against the specific bacteria that is commonly associated with acne. *(Always use carrier oil with the clove oil. Clove essential oil should not be directly applied to your skin)*

Supplements:

Vitamin A - This vitamin is readily available in many different food sources like cantaloupe, squash, carrots, sweet potatoes and dark leafy greens. Adding a vitamin A rich food into your daily diet will help support skin repair and immunity.

Lifestyle Tips:

Ditch Dairy and Use Gentle Products - Dairy products contain hormones that can disturb our own hormonal balance and stimulate our oil glands and pores. Opt for dairy and milk alternatives made from nuts or grains.

It is also important to use gentle, nutritive and natural products on your skin that won't further irritate or aggravate your acne. For a gentle, all-natural approach to skin care, you may benefit from my book, *Homemade Organic Skin & Body Care*, which includes lotions, cleansers, scrubs and body butters.

Body Odor and Perspiration:
Eliminating Toxins

Heavy or abnormal perspiration and the body odor associated with it are often considered a hygienic problem but in fact can be linked to metabolic toxins and hormonal fluctuations. Since overheating of our body may happen during fluctuations of estrogen, our body is trying to cool us by perspiring. If we are toxic inside the accompanying body odor will be worse. By using hormonal balancing techniques while addressing our inner health we can reduce body odor.

Herbs:
Tea Tree Essential Oil - This strong antibacterial herb will help reduce the unpleasant smells associated with perspiration. A few drops in water can be used as a wash.

Supplements:
Zinc & Magnesium - Studies have shown that by supplementing our diet with 15 mg of Zinc and Magnesium, body odor can be significantly reduced, and can also help regulate our adrenal, thyroid and insulin functions.

Lifestyle Tips:
Cut out Hard to Digest Foods and Take Steam Baths - When we eat foods that are difficult to digest, like rich fatty foods, red meat and dairy, our digestive system has to work hard to break down the food and in the process must release waste toxins. This toxic overload comes out during perspiration. Extra steam baths will help with this elimination process.

Withdrawal from Birth Control Pills:
Easing the Transition

When birth control pills are prescribed for symptoms like acne and heavy periods, they are not getting to the root of the problem: hormonal imbalance. So when you stop taking the pill, these symptoms are likely to come back without a holistic approach to hormones. Other symptoms related to withdrawing from contraceptives include the loss of water weight, mood swings, irregular periods, breast tenderness and appetite increases. Some women have reported positive symptoms including improved sleep, higher energy levels, clearer skin and lesser mood swings.

Herbs:
Vitex - By regulating our pituitary gland, which in turns supports our other glands, we can gently bring our system closer to balanced hormonal health. Take 250mg of the capsules daily.

Supplements:
Phytonutrients - These health-giving nutrients that are made up from what we know as 'superfoods' directly benefit our hormones by acting on a cellular level to improve bodily functions. Phytonutrients can be found in foods like kale, avocados, spinach and blueberries. Including these foods in your daily diet will help improve overall hormonal health.

Lifestyle Tips:
Cut Bad Fats and Include Good Fats - Eliminating processed vegetable oils, hydrogenated oils and margarines, and occasionally consuming unprocessed, whole-food fats (including nuts, seeds, coconut and olives) will assist in improved thyroid function.

Fibroids:
Minimizing their Effects

These non-cancerous growths in the uterus may appear during childbearing years, sometimes showing up only during pregnancy. Their level of growth can be associated with hormonal levels of estrogen and progesterone. At times they can cause no symptoms at all and other times they may cause heavier bleeding, pelvic pressure, frequent urination, constipation or backache.

Herbs:
Yellow Dock Root Capsules - This purifying herb stimulates bile, acts as a mild laxative and improves blood cell production. Also high in iron, Yellow Dock works as a general detoxifier for your system. 2 capsules, 3 times a day is standard.

Supplements:
High Fiber Foods with Phytoestrogens - The following foods all are high in fiber and gentle hormone balancers called phytoestrogens: Mangoes, apples, berries and grapes. Eat these foods in abundance to help with toxic waste removal and hormonal balance.

Lifestyle Tips:
Avoid Hormone Disruptors - Discussed previously in the introduction, hormone disruptors are chemicals that mimic hormones and throw off our hormonal balance when we are exposed to them. These chemicals can be found in commercial body care products, plastics, tobacco, etc.

Breast Cysts and Lumpiness:
Keeping them in Check

A scatter of small, fibrocystic lumps in the breasts often do not require treatment unless they are large and painful, and usually disappear after menopause. Their size is often relative to hormonal fluctuations and the real cause is unknown, though links to estrogen levels have been noted. Ensure to have a breast examination if you have any concerns or notice any new lumps.

Herbs:
Cranberry Juice Extract - Cranberry has one of the highest naturally occurring levels of iodine, an important nutrient. Iodine deficiency can lead to the formation of breast cysts. Rather than regular cranberry juice, use a teaspoon of unsweetened cranberry juice extract (sold in many natural food stores or online) which can be mixed with other all-fruit juices, like apple, as a daily tonic.

Supplements:
Vitamin E - Studies have revealed that supplementing with 400IU of Vitamin E daily may relieve the pain and tenderness of enlarged cysts.

Lifestyle Tips:
Supportive Bra and Heat - Underwire and too-tight bras have been linked with higher incidences of breast cysts. Wear supportive, breathable material (like cotton). Applying heat can relieve the tenderness of breast cysts.

PCOS and Fertility:
Harmonizing Your Hormones

Polycystic Ovary Syndrome is a condition in which many small cysts are present in the ovaries. It can cause symptoms such as weight gain, acne, increased facial hair and infrequent or irregular periods. PCOS represents the most common disorder responsible for malfunctioning ovaries causing infertility.

Herbs:
Rosemary - With its antioxidant, anti-inflammatory and immune boosting properties, rosemary, dried or fresh, works gently to balance the thyroid and eliminate excessive estrogen, common in women with PCOS. Use it in your cooked recipes, as a topping for roasted vegetables, or brew as a tea.

Supplements:
Vitamin D with Calcium - It has been reported that supplementing with Vitamin D and Calcium has been associated with higher rates of pregnancy and regular menstruation. Opt for a cruelty-free, plant-based Vitamin D supplement.

Lifestyle Tips:
Exercise and Plant Protein for Weight Loss - Most PCOS patients have been shown to be either obese or somewhat overweight. Embarking in a regular exercise program that includes aerobic activities, stretching or yoga and strength training will not only help with fat burning and weight loss, but also contributes to feelings

of self esteem and higher energy. Consuming a portion of plant-based proteins with your meals (such as beans, seeds or lentils) will assist in regulating insulin sensitivities associated with PCOS.

Endometriosis:
Natural Support

When the endometrium, the tissue that lines the uterus, grows outside the uterus it can cause pain, bowel problems, excessive bleeding and infertility. Surrounding tissues can also become irritated and menstrual symptoms may worsen. Though the exact reasons for endometriosis are unknown, bringing the body into hormonal balance may help the body to overcome this unnatural growth.

Herbs:
Milk Thistle - This detoxifying herb has the ability to break down and help eliminate excess estrogens. While cleansing the liver, milk thistle acts as an efficient body detoxifier and has a balancing effect on hormones. 70mg per day is the standard dose.

Supplements:
Selenium and Vitamin E - There's some evidence that endometriosis is caused or worsened by deficiencies in Selenium and Vitamin E. Take 400IU of Vitamin E and eat one brazil nut per day (which contains over 100% of daily recommended Selenium).

Lifestyle Tips:
Ditch Dairy and Drink Spring Water - Endometriosis can be exacerbated by an excess of estrogen which may worsened by the hormones found in milk and dairy. Municipal water contains the hormone disruptor, dioxin (from chlorine), so drinking only spring water or filtered water is recommended.

Cervical Dysplasia:
Encourage Extra Healing

This condition occurs when abnormal changes to cells appear on the surface of the cervix. It usually affects women ages 25-35, and if left untreated, may increase the risk of cancer. Cervical Dysplasia is often associated with Human Papillomavirus (HPV) and can be detected early with regular pap smears.

Herbs:
Vitex Tincture - To help your body regain hormonal balance, this herb enables hormonal balance to happen by supporting the endocrine system. It has been shown to effect positive results in cervical dysplasia. 30 drop per day of the tincture is suggested.

Supplements:
Folate & B12 - Deficiencies in Folate and B12 have been linked with higher rates of HPV infection. Taking a B-Complex vitamin daily will ensure you have the Folate, B12 and other B vitamins your body requires.

Lifestyle Tips:
Antioxidant Rich Foods & Safe Sex - Berries, cherries, tomatoes, squash and many other colorful, nutrient rich fruits and vegetables will boost your immunity and provide essential antioxidants for your body. By taking precautions to practice sex safe, you will be better able to protect yourself of HPV risks.

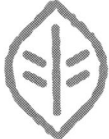

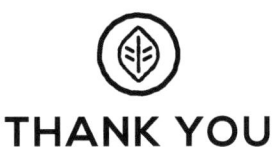

THANK YOU

Thank you for taking the time to read this comprehensive hormonal handbook. I hope you have gained a wealth of insight into our endocrine system and the importance of our hormones. We live in a world where unnecessary drugs, medications and invasive procedures are used to treat symptoms, instead of gently bringing our bodies back into balance. By implementing these simple, holistic tips into your life, you will reap the benefits of improved hormonal health – the *natural* way.

I wish you every success in your health and wellness journey!

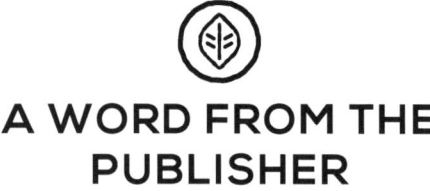

A WORD FROM THE PUBLISHER

Hi, I'm Carmen, a holistic health geek with a passion for health, herbalism, natural remedies, as well as whole-food and plant-based lifestyles. After resolving various health issues I have struggled with for many years, I aim to inspire and help improve your health and longevity by sharing the tireless hours of research and valuable information I have discovered throughout my journey. Through the power of nutrition and lifestyle, with an evidence-based approach, I believe you can achieve your health and wellness goals.

If you enjoyed this book, I would love to hear how it has benefited you and invite you to leave a short review on Amazon - your valuable feedback is always appreciated!

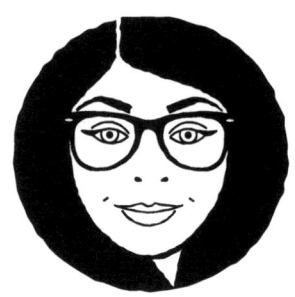

You are invited to to join our **Free Book Club** *mailing list. Sign up via our website to receive* **special offers** *and* **free for a limited time** *Health & Wellness eBooks!*

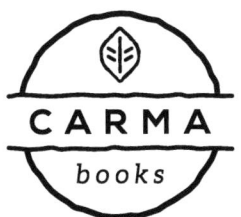

'A conscious approach to health & wellness'

carmabooks.com

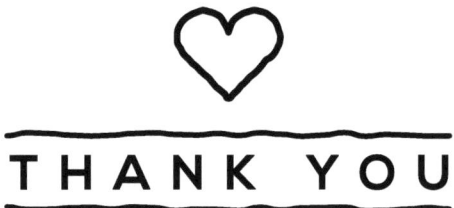

Printed in Poland
by Amazon Fulfillment
Poland Sp. z o.o., Wrocław